Chakra For Beginners

Chakra Balancing

April Stone

You agree that by continuing to read this book, where appropriate and/or necessary, you shall consult a professional (including but not limited to your doctor, attorney, or financial advisor or such other advisor as needed) before using any of the suggested remedies, techniques, or information in this book.

ISBN: 1547210869

ISBN-13: 978-1547210862

CONTENTS

What are chakras?

You are energy. All life is made of energy.

You may have heard through modern science of all the different types of bodily systems within you, such as the nervous system and the immune system. These of course are exceptionally important in the human body for keeping us safe and well. But what about the energy system?

Intertwined with physical and mental wellbeing, energy is arguably one of the most important aspects of life. It courses through everything, impacting nature in every conceivable way. For a human it can affect you physically, through such things as organ function, the immune system, and even sex drive, as well as mentally through things like your emotions, your mental clarity, and your thought processes. You are full of energy, shaping your every action and reaction.

At certain points within you, there are places where this energy is the most active—known as energy centers. When your energy centers function at the highest level, you are kept mentally, emotionally, physically, and spiritually balanced. These energy centers have come to be known as chakras.

Defining the chakras

Meaning "wheel" or "disc", chakras can be thought of as little spinning, colored wheels inside the human body, their power constantly flowing and ebbing inside of you, able to disperse and absorb life-energy (also known prana)—that is, the energy of the universe. Briefly, from the base of the spine, they are the Root (1st) chakra; the Sacral (2nd) chakra in the lower abdomen; the Solar Plexus (3rd) chakra in the upper abdomen; the Heart (4th) chakra in the center of the chest; the Throat (5th) chakra in the throat; the Third Eye (6th) chakra between the eyes; and the Crown (7th) chakra at the top of the head. There are also twenty-one minor chakras distributed over the body, and within these are grouped ten bilateral minor chakras.

Each chakra works both independently and together in order to help make us balanced human beings. Yogic teachings from India give the seven major chakras specific qualities, such as color (originating from the spectrum of light), elements (air, water, earth, etc.), and body sense (touching, smelling, tasting, etc.). You can think of these energy centers as being connected vertically by a power line; this power line constantly emptying and absorbing prana, which ebbs, flows and spreads out from the center of your body to your limbs, and the very tips of your fingers and toes. The Vajrayana system states that the power line starts at the Third Eye, then curves up to the top of the head, and back down to the lower body.

The chakras work like a power grid, gathering energy before expelling just the right amount through the electrical network (pathways, also known as nades) inside of you. Simply through spinning, the chakras draw in prana, convert energy and expel it through the nades to reach all parts of your body, and in the process keep the energies in perfect harmony.When working in harmony; the chakras provide the perfect balance of energies, leading to a healthy mind, healthy body, spiritual freedom and the ultimate level of inner peace. This allows the optimal setting for meditation, whether that be meditation, how you might picture it, or a more active form, such as practicing yoga. Through meditation in conjunction with the utilization of the chakras, you can achieve or enhance dream yoga or lucid dreaming.

Chakras can be seen, but only through specialist equipment (Kirlian photography) or to individuals who are gifted with having the ability to perceive chakras with the naked eye. They do this by seeing the aura that chakras project around us.

Evolution of the chakras

Chakras have been a concept since ancient times. The original definition of "chakra" being "wheel" is in reference to chakravartins, a term from ancient India that was used to refer to the ultimate universal ruler—one who is peaceful, ethical, compassionate and benevolent to all the world and its people. Chakravartins were described as having a spinning, lit-up golden disk in front of their chests, like chakras, perhaps due to powerful Solar Plexus chakras.

The first recordings of chakras that we know of are in theYogatattva Upanishad and Brahma Upanishad — the Upanishads being a collection of ancient texts of a religious and philosophical nature originating from India, most likely in 800BC to 500BC, though historians believe that the concept of chakras reaches as far back as 1500BC and possibly recorded from established oral tradition. Since these writings; the concept of the chakras has developed into a more refined system — being adapted into Tibetan Buddhism and the now well-used Tantric Shakta theory. It is the Tantric Shakta theory that is most prevalent today, due to the Sat-Cakra-Nirupana, written in 1577, and the 10th century book Padaka-Pancaka. These books were translated in to English by the prominent British writer, Sir John Woodroffe under the pseudonym Arthur Avalon, in the book The Serpent Power, which was published in 1919. This allowed the west to first understand the concept of chakras. Along with another text for the 10th century,

Gorakshashatakam, the Sat-Cakra-Nirupana and the Padaka-Pancaka form the basis of how we understand chakras today. The book is both very comprehensive and quite complicated, and has now developed into the generally-accepted Western view on chakras, demonstrated by C. W. Leadbeater in the 1927 book The Chakras.

In modern society, many cultures have taken the concept of chakras, or something similar, and integrated it into all types of holistic healing. Some cultures have even developed their own theories independently using similar thought processes. Most notably, the Chinese concept of "chi" references the same type of cosmic energy that prana refers to. Also, some thinkers today propose that the chakras possess a physical form as well as a spiritual form. Some have postulated the position of the six lower chakras match the position of some major nerve plexuses along the spinal cord. Others have suggested they could be linked to the endocrine glands or the pineal gland. It was even suggested by 20th century writer Rudolf Steiner that the chakra system is evolving with us; different from how they were in ancient times and our modern bodies, but these theories are yet to be proven.

The Chakras are becoming and increasing popular concept, and are a part of cultures all over the world. Balancing chakras, which is what this book will take you through, is now becoming more increasingly common as a form of alternative treatment. When thirty years ago chakras had little credibility, more people are turning to this system to help themselves. In the 21st century, you won't be too hard-pushed to find an expert of chakra healing in your city, or even a course to help you understand the chakras and how to heal them through varying techniques. Part of a happy and fulfilled life is making sure your chakras are working perfectly and are remaining in balance.

You are energy, and it is a natural process to make sure that this energy is working in perfect balance to be of maximum benefit to you, your body, your mind, your dreams, your loved ones, your life, and your future as you want it.

The power of balancing your chakras

Keeping your chakras balanced is crucial to self-satisfaction and spiritual development. As each chakra is tied to a different aspect of your physical, mental and spiritual self, any imbalance in these can cause hugely detrimental effects. When they are balanced, you'll also reap the rewards of this with notable enhancements in your mind, body and soul.

Benefits of keeping your chakras balanced

Balancing chakras has long been tied to enhancing meditation. Meditative contemplation opens you up, aiding you in enhancing your psychic and spiritual awareness, giving you inner peace, and a helping you to attain general self-satisfaction in your life. Meditation always works best when you have complete mental, emotional, spiritual, and physical balance.

Physically, balancing your chakras can help strengthen the immune system, giving it health and power in order to help stave off illnesses. This is especially beneficial, as these illnesses bring with them negative energies, emotions, and physical feelings. Balancing your chakras can also help with enhancing your sex drive.

Chakra balancing will also significantly help you when it comes to emotions. When all is balanced, you will have complete control over your emotions and be able to release them in a healthy, positive way, and not in a destructive manner that causes problems with you and the people that surround you. You could also alleviate boredom by helping your mind to inject enthusiasm and passion into the most mundane tasks, such as a boring work assignment or an otherwise unwanted errand. You can become more confident when speaking in public, and achieve better communication with people in general. This leads to more positive effects on your life in all aspects.

You can also enhance your relationships with the people close to you through stronger love and healthier connections with them, while making you better at forgiving, and increase your patience. No matter where you are in your relationship, you can experience more love and tolerance for the people that surround you. Past grievances can be forgotten, and your relationship with them can burn brighter than before.

Balancing your chakras can also turn weaknesses into strengths, and help to alleviate negative behavior patterns. There are many behaviors that could be perceived as negative, depending on the activity or situation—you could lack the ability to take the initiative in a challenging situation, you could be an otherwise irresponsible or lazy person, or you could follow patterns of aggression in both physical and mental violence. This physical and mental violence could be against you or others, and can manifest in scary ways. You could be implementing negative behavior patterns into your everyday life, through work practices and general habits, which are allowed to continually reinforce themselves and affect you directly. Chakra balancing can help to remedy these negative behaviors and behaviors like these into much more positive ones.

Not only can it help with the above kinds of negative behaviors, but also negative mental patterns. A lack of self-confidence, self-worth and self-love can be a constant fight in the struggle to live how you want to, and you may find yourself performing repetitive negative behaviors that only serve to increase feelings of self-loathing in perpetual destruction. Through balancing your chakras, these negative behaviors can be tackled through enhancing your own stability and enabling you to accept yourself as you are. You won't be afraid to express yourself, and this will result in higher self-confidence, leading to a greater sense of self-worth. Personal integrity is the key to success, and chakra balancing can help you to edge nearer to total self-mastery, which could be considered as the ultimate goal. Chakra balancing can dramatically increase your zest for life, leading to you garnering greater pleasure from life in general, and to help you to enjoy living in the present, and not constantly in want of the future.

This increased zest for life can lead to enhanced will and drive, steering you to do what you want by helping you to make clear, meaningful choices where the end goals are clear to you. This enhanced will and drive can also lead to more creativity and greater inspiration. You can increase your focus and help your intuition, leading to greater inner wisdom. This in turn can help you to become aware of your life path, and greatly increase your chances of getting there through making yourself open to all fortunes. This can lead to luck turning in your favor. Maybe you can earn more money, or a promotion at work, or otherwise guide an opportunity towards you that you wouldn't have otherwise been able to see.

Balancing the chakras when used in conjunction with other healing techniques such as modern medicine can lead to great physical, mental and spiritual benefits.

The bad effects of out of balance chakras

If you are confronted by a physical, emotional, mental or spiritual problem, balancing your chakras is a positive step in overcoming these issues. When chakras are blocked or unclean, they can lead to negative effects in the areas they control. These negative effects and manifest in physical, emotional and mental form, which can be very dangerous.

Physically, you may find yourself in pain, particularly headaches and in the lower back. You could be experiencing disorders of the skin, the heart, digestive, immune or nervous systems, or even the thyroid or bladder. You could experience breathing issues or problems with the teeth. You could also find yourself having a low sex drive, or poor circulation. All of these conditions can lead to potentially serious long-term physical problems.

Emotionally, you may find yourself having low self-esteem, leading to poor decisions and in turn a low sense of self-worth. You could find yourself craving so much approval that when that need is inevitably not fulfilled, it could evolve into deeper problems such as self-abuse or the habitual abusing of others, as well as addictions, moodiness and depression. You may find yourself constantly missing your goals through a lack of willpower and strength, leading to anger, bitterness, resentment, deep sadness, and jealousy for those who seem to be achieving their ambitions before you have achieved yours. You could also close your heart, and isolate yourself from others, excluding yourself from them, making you lonely and socially unfulfilled.

Mentally, imbalanced chakras could cause you to be indecisive whilst being overly-analytical. You may examine situations at length, and unconsciously choose the option that will be the most self-sabotaging. You could find yourself unable to express yourself adequately in words through unclear communication and being scattered and forgetful, leading to increasing frustration and rising self-hatred, as well as hatred for others. Frequent boredom can also be a problem, as well as a general apathy for your hobbies, your close ones, your job, or life in general. Your creativity could be seriously depressed, leading to a lack of imagination. This can come from the constant sapping of motivation and drive.

You could find yourself becoming increasingly aggressive, which could manifest in a dogmatic approach in communication, passing harsh judgement or criticism of others or the things that others create. You could also find yourself becoming increasingly materialistic and approaching everything in life through your own ego. Egotistical decisions will be made, creating social, mental and physical problems, as you become insecure and in want of a quick fix, however it comes. A general disconnection to life reality is also a sign of imbalanced chakras, as you retreat into yourself and become increasingly disconnected from the world around you.

If you are confronted by a physical, emotional, mental or spiritual problem, balancing your chakras will give you a greater ability to heal these problems faster and to a stronger degree. Without this balance, you could become trapped in a never-ending cycle of self-sabotage, only serving through you deeper into a hole that you can't get out of.

The seven chakras

As mentioned, there are seven main chakras through the body, beginning at the base of the spine, placed intermittently up to the top of the head. Each chakra has a certain location, symbol, color and area that it influences in the body.

The Root (or Base) Chakra

The Root chakra is the crucial building block for the rest of our chakra system. It is at the base of the spine. Being at the base, it is the foundation on which the rest of the chakras lay, and it is the very center of our life force. In Sanskrit, this chakra is known as "muladhara", meaning "root" (mula) and "support/base" (adhara).

It is associated both with the element of earth and the color red, however, traditionally this chakra can also be linked to gold or yellow, as this is the color of the earth element. Red color in the spectrum of the chakras represents our instinct, as well as vitality and strength in all senses of the word. Its symbol is a lotus flower with four petals, and it is often depicted as a circle containing a triangle pointing downwards. This triangle is representative of our bodies connecting with the earth and grounding us within nature.

Being at the base of the spine, physically, it is affiliated with the first three vertebrae, the perineum, and the pelvis, as well as the body's adrenaline control centers, our blood, our spine and our reproductive organs. Mentally, it deals with basic instincts and primal-level functions, such as the need to feel safe and secure; the will to survive; the need to find shelter, eat and sleep; and primal traits associated with our physical identity or our physicality. Root chakra is the very center of our being, and the base on which we build our lives.

The Sacral Chakra

The Sacral chakra is responsible for our joie de vivre. The Sacral chakra has a different location according to different chakra systems, but most commonly it is believed that it lies three inches under our navel and in line with the lumbar vertebrae, sitting at the very core of our being. In Sanskrit, it is called "syadisthana", which means the "dwelling place" or "your own place".

The Sacral chakra is linked to with the water element, and is most commonly associated with the color orange, which is usually quite transparent and translucent. However, as it is joined with the water element, it can also be associated with light blue, or, very rarely, even white. Orange represents emotions and creativity. The Sacral chakra's symbol is a flower with six petals, inside containing a circle with a crescent moon. The circle itself represents the Sacral chakra's associated element, water, and the Moon, usually silver, is the link between the Moon and the water element. This is the association of the Moon and emotions, as well as the Moon having links to the reproductive system in women.

Physically, it is associated with the lymphatic system of the kidneys, and the reproductive organs, such as the ovaries, testes and the uterus. Mentally, the Sacral chakra fuels creativity, energy, sex drive, and confidence, as well as being part of our connection with others. It is all that is pleasant in life.

The Solar Plexus (or Navel) Chakra

The Solar Plexus chakra is responsible for our willpower and assertiveness. It is commonly accepted to be located in the diaphragm, although some traditions are not so restrictive with its location, and place it more loosely around the navel. In Sanskrit, it is known as "manipura", meaning "city of jewels". It can also be known as the nabhi ("navel") or the "power chakra".

The Solar Plexus chakra is combined with the element of fire, however, some modern interpretations now link it with air. Its associated color is yellow, or a yellow-red, due to its association with fire. In chakra color meaning, yellow is linked to intellect. The Solar Plexus' chakra symbol is a flower with ten petals, and inside the circle a downward-pointing triangle. The triangle is representative of the element of fire and the power of transformation, such as fire can burn and provide fuel, with which we can propel ourselves forward.

Physically, it correlates with the central nervous system, the pancreas, the digestive system (such as our intestines or stomach), the liver, the pancreas, and the metabolic system (involved in how we obtain energy from the food we eat). Mentally, it is all that is our drive. It's self-confidence and willpower, helping us to take control of our lives and make decisions that lead to achieving our goals. It's also intelligence and clarity of thought, and helps invoke personal identity through aiding us to form beliefs and opinions personal to us, resulting in us achieving independence.

The Heart Chakra

As you might expect, the Heart chakra is essential to love, connection, and beauty. It is located, importantly, not where the human heart is, but in the center of the chest. This chakra exists in multiple dimensions—at the front, it passes through the center of the chest, and at the back it passes through the shoulder blades. In Sanskrit, it is "anahata" ("unstruck"). This is also known as "hritpankaja" ("heart lotus").

This particular chakra is joined with the air element, associating it with space, breadth, balance and connection. When usually you might think of love as pink, the Heart chakra is more commonly related to the color green. The reason you may think of the heart as pink is due to the color of the aura is emits; usually seen as pink. Green is depicted as being the color of balance, serenity and general healing. The Heart's chakra symbol is a flower with twelve petals, with both an upward-facing triangle and a downward-facing triangle interlocked, which form a star shape. These triangles arranged together in this way are the balance of gender, matter and spirit.

Physically, the Heart chakra is linked with things in the region it is placed, such as the lungs and the cardiac system, and also the immune system and hormones through its connection with the thymus gland. Mentally, it is best summed up by the words "love" and "connection". It perpetuates unconditional love for both others and ourselves, and enhances our compassion, forgiveness, and empathy for others, allowing us to forge stronger and healthier relationships. When we're faced with bad circumstances, it can aid in grieving and overcoming them. It aids our appreciation of beauty in all things and promotes general harmony with those around us.

The Throat Chakra

The Throat chakra is the link between the body and the head, and as such can be a "bottleneck" for energies in the Heart chakra, and also a good point to start when balancing chakras. This is the chakra for communication, and connection with the spirit. It is located at the bottom of the throat, where the clavicles meet to form the V-shape, but also has associations with the mouth, in the jaw, palette and tongue, and also the neck and shoulders. Like the Heart chakra, it is also multi-dimensional, and extends to come out of the throat at the front at an upwards angle. In Sanskrit, it is called "vishuddha" ("pure").

The Throat chakra's element is sound (which can also be known as ether). It relates to all matters involving sound, particularly speech. Its color is usually blue, but the energy in the Throat chakra aura can also be purple. Blue in the chakra color system associated with communication, the serenity of the soul, and complete purification. The Throat chakra's symbol is a flower with sixteen petals, inside of which is a circle containing a downward-facing triangle, with another circle inside the triangle. The downward-facing triangle is related to learning, as the sides slope up to channel this learning into enlightenment.

Physically, the Throat chakra, as mentioned above,

connects with all parts of the body in its region, such as the shoulders, the mouth, and the ears. It is also strongly associated with the thyroid, which helps to maintain growth, temperature and metabolism of the human body. Mentally, it is the chakra that is crucial for good communication in any form, whether that be verbal through language, or non-verbal through expressions and movement. It's a chakra that helps us to express ourselves as we want to be seen, by aiding us in accurately and competently changing creative ideas into reality—through this, the Throat chakra is linked very closely with the Sacral chakra. It is also a chakra that is hugely instrumental in connecting with the spirit.

The Third Eye (or Brow) Chakra

The Third Eye chakra represents foresight, imagination, and good intuition. It is located between your eyebrows both horizontally and vertically—often misunderstood to be in the center of the forehead—and it is behind the eyes. In Sanskrit, it is known as "ajna" ("command" or "perceiving").

This chakra's element is the "supreme element", which simply means all of the elements put together, but its element has also been described as being light, or even time. Its associated color is indigo, which is symbolic of awareness and consciousness. However, this chakra is not really about the color, but rather how luminescent that color is. The symbol is a flower with a large petal on either side, and the flower contains a downward-facing triangle. The downward-facing triangle, as in the Throat chakra, is a channel of wisdom, from gathering the information to channeling it up into enlightenment.

Physically, the chakra is connected with the pineal gland, which maintains biorhythms, such as the circadian rhythm (sleep cycle), as well the left eye, the ears, and the nose. Mentally, as well as physically being involved in vision, it is also crucial to our inner vision. It increases our abilities of inner perception to detect subtle energy movements. Psychic abilities come through the Third Eye, and it gives us good insight and higher wisdom. Additionally, it can give us more inspiration and creativity.

The Crown Chakra

The Crown chakra is the chakra that allows us into states of higher consciousness. It is located at the very top of the head, or sometimes is described as being slightly above the head. The reason it is called the Crown chakra is due to how the chakra sits on the head in the way a crown does. This chakra has a particular connection with the Root chakra, as these chakras sit on opposite ends of the chakra system. In Sanskrit, the Crown chakra is known as, "sahasrara", generally translated as "thousand petals".

The Crown chakra's element is cosmic energy, or sometimes thought. This is prana, and the energy then runs through the chakra system. It is identified with the color violet, which is the color of cosmic consciousness, and is about spirituality and healing. Sometimes this chakra links to the color white and its field of aura can be gold, or even clear. The symbol for the Crown chakra is a circle in a thousand petals, and because of how it looks, it is sometimes associated with the Full Moon.

Physically, due to its placement, it is associated with the endocrine system, as it is linked with the hypothalamus and the pituitary gland. It is also related to the brain and the central nervous system, and the right eye. Mentally, the Crown is crucial to consciousness and awareness, helping us to achieve wisdom and to fathom what is sacred. It helps us to forge a connection with the formless, and provides us with realization. It gives us ecstasy, and a greater presence. The Crown chakra provides us with the awareness to transcend our limitations, with clarity and wisdom. It can be a gateway to your higher self.

Why your chakras are out of balance.

If you are feeling out of kilter, it is more than likely to be caused by an imbalanced chakra. Whether you're finding it hard to sleep, if you have lower back pain, if you are having problems communicating with people, these are all signs that a chakra is not balanced.

Sometimes life can take dramatic twists and turns, and the chakras can become blocked. This causes the other chakras to compensate, showing up as overactive (so the traits they bring are amplified into levels you cannot cope with) or underactive (where these feelings are not enough). Whether overactive or underactive, they can greatly affect you and your day-to-day life.

There are many physical, mental, emotional, and

even spiritual reasons manifestations of imbalanced chakras, and fortunately, you can identify symptoms and match them to a chakra in order to know where the issue resides.

Root (or Base) Imbalance

As discussed, the Root chakra is associated with your basic instincts and actions—self-preservation. When this chakra is working, you will feel safe, secure, and comfortable in your life and your instincts

Mentally

An imbalance in this chakra results in a general feeling of insecurity, and not being safe. This over amplified need for security can put others basics survival needs in jeopardy.

Worrying about work/money/providing basic needs: Feeling inadequate in providing basic needs and being in a constant survival mode, potentially resulting in stress, anxiety, and depression. This is a symptom of underactivity.

Desire to satisfy own needs and wants: The need to satisfy your own desires and wants, and not others, leading to poor relationships. This is a sign of overactivity.

Being materialistic: To compensate for your lack of security, you could find yourself buying goods to please yourself. This can result in over-inflated self-esteem, all stemming from an overactivity of the Root chakra.

Resistance to change: If you're finding you are resisting a change in your life, this is usually a sign of overactivity.

Eating disorders: A sign of underactivity, any eating disorder is an effect of a problem in basic instincts provided by this chakra.

Physically

When imbalanced, basics functions of the body can go awry, such as eating, sleeping, blood, and the skeleton. Due to its placement, conditions of the legs and feet are also common.

Fatigue

Frequent urinating

Cold feet and hands resulting from bad circulation

High/low blood pressure

Suppressed immune system

Bone problems

Digestion problems

Leg, hip, and feet problems

Sacral Imbalance

Associated with your pleasures in life, when working, your Sacral chakra offers pleasure, enhancing sexual experiences and emotional connections.

Mentally

Imbalance can cause problems in connecting with those around you. The satisfaction you take from pleasures in life could be over realized or under-realized, with disastrous consequences.

Poor relationships: Resulting from overly-dominant relationships, an inability to emotionally connect with others, stiffness, and a constant fear of betrayal. This results in poor, short, and potentially abusive relationships.

No enthusiasm for life: As the Sacral chakra is about pleasure, being unable to gain pleasure from life is a sign of it being severely underactive.

Inability to overcome addictions: Any overactivity in the Sacral chakra can result in the need to gain high pleasure hits, which results in addiction that can be hard to beat.

Inability to enjoy sex: The center of your sexual drive, any underactivity will mean gaining little or no pleasure from sexual experiences.

Overemotional: Overactivity in the Sacral chakra can lead you to emotionally overreacting, and you can have an addiction to drama.

Physically

With its strong connection to the reproductive system, any problem in this area is connected to the Sacral chakra. As per its location, any lower back, bowel, or kidney problem is also connected.

Irregular menstrual cycles

Reproductive issues

Kidney problems

Irritable Bowel Syndrome

Back and joint pain

Solar Plexus imbalance

The Solar Plexus is about control, and when working helps you to control your emotions and mind, and your life.

Mentally

Your drive and love of yourself may increase or decrease to troublesome proportions. You may find yourself having a need to be constantly praised, or a fear of confronting others.

Low self-esteem: Generally feeling as though you're worthless and powerless in the course of your life is a sign of underactivity in the Solar Plexus chakra.

Fear of other's opinions: Needing to feel self-worth stems this symptom of an underactive Solar Plexus chakra.

Aggressive and controlling: An overactive Solar Plexus chakra can result in domineering and over-critical behavior towards others.

Easy to use: Feelings of being passive and timid are a sign of underactivity, which will allow others to take advantage of you.

Constant pessimism: Feeling pessimistic and down on your luck results from Solar Plexus underactivity.

Physically

This chakra is closely associated with the stomach area, so illnesses relating to food intake are connected.

Fatigue

High blood pressure

Stomach problems

Pancreas problems

Food cravings

Diabetes

Gluten intolerance

Heart Imbalance

The Heart chakra is all about love. When this chakra is balanced, it helps your capability to forgive, accept, and love all those around you.

Mentally

When this chakra is out of balance, your need to be loved can go haywire, resulting in either stifling relationships or being completely closed emotionally.

Overly loving: From overactivity of the Chakra, your need for love can be increased, leading to problems of being "clingy" or "suffocating" of your partner.

Easy to use: As a result of overactivity, you could find yourself saying "yes" to anything others ask or tell you to do. You could lack any boundaries and allow people to walk all over you.

Closed emotions: An underactive Heart chakra stunts your ability to feel. You may find yourself becoming very guarded, distant and cold, which in turn is feeling loneliness.

Need for acceptance: Your need for love in overactivity of this chakra can lead to you trying desperately to be accepted, as well as being on the constant lookout for praise and rewards.

Physically

The Heart chakra's area in the body can tell you whether it needs balancing, as it dominates the chest and the upper back. It is also closely linked to skin problems, such as acne or rashes.

Skin problems

Upper back and shoulder problems

Lung problems

Heart problems

Pain in the arms and wrists

Breast problems

Throat Imbalance

Communication is the key in the Throat chakra. When balanced, this chakra allows you to communicate both verbally and non-verbally with ease.

Mentally

The Throat chakra's role in communication means that when imbalanced, you could either become overly verbal or completely unable to communicate your ideas.

Overly introversive: With underactivity of this chakra comes excessive shyness. You could be quiet and unconfident, and feel as though you cannot properly articulate yourself from a fear of not saying things 'correctly'.

Poor communication: In opposition with the above,

with an overactive chakra you can become overly verbal. You can become too talkative, too critical, and very condescending with your inability to control your communication.

Powerlessness: From underactivity, with a lack of good communication skills and the inability to speak up, you will find it easier just to follow people, resulting in a lack of power.

Low confidence: When underactive, you become hyper-aware that your inability to communicate can result in bad reactions. You became fearful of judgment and others rejecting you, so your confidence will be very low.

Physically

The Throat chakra is so closely linked to the mouth and throat that problems in this area are to do with its imbalance. It can also be linked to the ears and the very top of the torso.

Throat problems

Mouth problems

Ear infections

Neck and shoulder problems

Third Eye Imbalance

The Third Eye is imagination, foresight, and intuition. When in balance, this chakra allows clarity of thought and correct anticipation.

Mentally

Out of balance, this chakra can cause problems in focused and self-reflection. You'll be unable to trust yourself, confused in complex situations and find yourself constantly drifting.

Lack of ability in self-reflection: You will be unable to reflect on yourself when this chakra is overactive. You'll have a lack of commitment to projects and confidence problems, as you won't feel like you can trust your reasoning and your inner voice.

Daydreaming: Excessive daydreaming is a symptom of an overactive Third Eye chakra. You could feel as though you're living in kind of fantasy world, and constantly find yourself disconnected from reality.

Confusion: It is quick to confuse someone with an underactive Third Eye chakra. You'll struggle to comprehend things, as you'll be unable to see subtext or the points of view of other people.

Overly-stoic: From underactivity, the inability to interpret others can make you very rigid in your thinking, and you could rely on authority too much while being closed off to new ideas.

Physically

The Third Eye is connected to most problems involving the upper part of your head, including your ears, your sinuses, and your eyes.

Headaches

Vision problems

Ear problems

Sinus problems

Crown Imbalance

The Crown chakra provides wisdom and presence. It allows you to evolve to higher consciousness and connect with cosmic energy.

Mentally

When imbalanced, your head and your body can become disconnected from one another. You will find it hard to connect with your spirit, learn new things and let go of negative emotions.

Cannot learn: You could find yourself unable to analyze new information, either as learning or in your surroundings. From an underactive crown, this can result in feeling very confused. Overthinking: too many thoughts you can't process, can't switch brain off (over)

Feeling disconnected: With your Crown chakra being underactive, you could find yourself feeling disconnected from the world around you, and cause you to feel very insignificant.

Depression and anxiety: This results from overactivity of this chakra. You might find yourself unable to let go of events. You could also be feeling unsatisfied in life.

Unable to control emotions: Here, an overactivity of the Crown chakra causes an inability in controlling emotions, and they may begin to take over your life.

Physically

Overactivity can enhance the senses in your head to uncomfortable proportions, and make you have trouble emotionally and even cause lack of sleep.

Headache/Migraine

Insomnia

Mood swings

Dizziness

Increased sensitivity to vision and sound

How to begin healing your chakra

Determining whether you have a damaged chakra comes down to whether you're feeling unlike your normal self. Any kind of feeling or lack of feeling, mental or physical, points to an imbalance, and the chakra causing the problem can be identified according to the type of problem and its location.

Root: Are you worried about money, or basic needs and instincts? Having problems with blood or bones?

Sacral: Are you having problems in relationships, or in your reproductive system?

Solar Plexus: Do you have low self-esteem, or feel emotionally weak? Is there a problem relating to the stomach area of the body?

Heart: Are you finding it hard to love and trust someone? Do you have a skin problem, or a problem related to the chest?

Throat: Do you have an issue when you speak to others? Do you have a physical problem with the mouth and throat?

Third Eye: Are you having trouble thinking clearly, or find yourself constantly in a daydream? Are you having headaches and eye problems?

Crown: Find it hard to let go of negative emotions, or having issues connecting? Are your senses overly acute?

Different chakras may be imbalanced at the same time. According to the problem you are having and where you are experiencing it; you can narrow it down and determine which chakras are imbalanced. Once identified, you can begin to help redress that balance.

Immediate Treatment for Imbalanced Chakras

When starting on the journey to balancing your chakras, after identifying which chakra may be imbalanced, there is another thing to consider —the connection between the chakras is strong, so once the imbalanced chakra has been identified, you should also consider working on its neighboring chakras, as they could be affected by the imbalance. When a particular chakra is overactive or underactive, this disrupts the flow of prana throughout the entire chakra system.

Each chakra has its own attachment to certain activities. Performing these activities can help to heal your chakra and redress the balance. Here are some activities you can do at this exact moment without any preparation.

Root Chakra

Stand up and breathe. It may seem so simple, but this is the first step to helping redress that imbalance. Right now, stand with your upper half relaxed, and breathe for a while.

Have a wash. Either by a shower or a bath with "earthly" aromatic oils (e.g. cedar, cypress, clove). As you do this, be sure to remain aware of your physical body, and all the movements it does.

Go for a walk. Head outside. This chakra is so connected with the Earth that simply going for a walk can help it. Reconnect with nature. Be aware of your movement and your breath as you take each stride. Don't be afraid to slip off your shoes and stomp on the ground, and feel the grass between your toes.

Work in the garden. It's the connection with nature we desire. Do you have a garden? If so, weed, or plant something. You want the mud of the Earth on your hands and clothes.

Utilize red. Red is the associated color of this

chakra. Eat red food, and gaze at anything you have near you in the color red, put on any red clothes you have.

Dance. Free, uninhibited movement either with people or by yourself is a connection to your natural self and it allows you to connect with the Earth. You don't have to have music. Get up now, and let your natural instincts control your flow. Move the hips.

Have a pedicure. The Root chakra's connected to the feet means that taking care of your feet offers great benefits. If you cannot have a pedicure at this moment then try washing your feet or painting your toenails. Massage your feet. Just make sure they are taken care of.

Sacral Chakra

Dance. As well as being good for your Root chakra, dancing is great for your Sacral. The freedom of body movement helps the Sacral chakra energy to flow.

Watch romantic films. Particularly watch romcoms. If your partner is with you, snuggle up and watch something loving and funny together.

Be creative. What do you feel like creating? Create something out of nothing, in whatever medium you choose. Don't worry if the end result's good or not — it's the creative process that is the most healing. This will soothe and nurture an imbalanced Sacral chakra.

Laugh. Find something to make you laugh right now, whether that be a friend, an online video, or something on television.

Find pleasing scents. The Sacral is pleasure, and powerful smells are of great benefit. If you have aromatic oils or herbs, then use them, or simply head outside, smell a flower, and take in the pleasant aroma.

Utilize orange. Orange is the color of this chakra, so eat orange food, wear orange clothes, or find orange things you have to surround yourself with.

Let go of your feelings. Bottling up emotions is to this chakra's detriment. Find an understanding friend to talk to, or keep a journal; let these emotions out, now.

Solar Plexus Chakra

Sit in the sun. If the sun is out at the moment, bask in the sun for twenty minutes. You can help destroy any negativity that is causing this chakra to be imbalanced.

Utilize yellow. Yellow is associated with this chakra. Eating yellow food, wearing yellow clothes and finding yellow objects to surround yourself with will all help.

Exercise. Quickly do some exercises that connect with this Chakra's location. Movement of the body is always positive.

Do what you've been meaning to. Maybe you've always wanted to try baking a cake, or perhaps the house needs hoovering. No matter the task, whether creative or a chore, do it to help balance your Solar Plexus.

Positive reinforcement. Say this sentence out loud, "I am always brilliant". What did you think when you said it? If you catch yourself thinking negatively about yourself, then stop. Think about those negativities. How could they be positive? Do they really apply to you?

Heart Chakra

Tell your reflection "I love you". Find a mirror and take some time to gaze at your reflection, and let it know that you love it. By this, you can start to love yourself again.

Connect with children. The unconditional love we feel towards a baby or child is part of this chakra, and in turn, children have extraordinarily powerful Heart chakra energy. If you have a friend with a child, call them and visit them as soon as you can, and take some time to hold and connect with the young one.

Forgive others. Either by confronting the person you feel has wronged you, or by writing down what you want to say and burning it. Forgiveness is part of this chakra, so you must take positive steps to forgive others, and yourself.

Utilize green or pink. As mentioned, this chakra is green, but is also associated with the color pink. Clothes, objects or foods of these colors will both have a great effect.

Be thankful. Take this moment to think about everything in your life that you are thankful for. Friends, job, family, the store assistant who took the time to make sure you had the right product, and smiled whilst doing it. Big things or little things, being thankful is hugely beneficial to this chakra.

Do what you love doing. If you have a particular hobby that you can do on your own, get up now and do it. If possible, schedule this hour to do this hobby without interruption, as often as you possibly can.

Throat Chakra

Sing. It doesn't matter whether you can sing or not. Fill your lungs, open your mouth and sing your favorite songs. Even humming is hugely beneficial, if you don't currently feel confident enough to sing. Sing absolutely anywhere!

Drink water. Get a glass of water, now. Keep the throat lubricated with water, making sure the Throat chakra is clear.

Exercise your neck. This is the location of this chakra, so start taking care of it right now by doing some slow rotations and turns of your neck, stretching and exercising it.

Utilize blue. With blue being the color of this chakra, blue foods, blue clothes, and blue objects are all beneficial.

Talk to yourself. Don't be afraid to look in the mirror and have a positive conversation with yourself. Any form of vocalization is effective with this chakra.

Third Eye Chakra

Access your Third Eye. The Third Eye is in the center of your head, behind your eyes. Take a second. Close your eyes, and imagine looking through the Third Eye. Accept whatever you see. Explore it as far as you can.

Utilize purple. Connected with purple, this chakra loves purple foods, purple clothes, and purple objects around you.

Trust yourself. When your Third Eye chakra is having problems, it can seem as though you can't trust your own intuition. Chances are you are having a dilemma at this moment. What is your gut feeling about this situation? Go with it. When it turns out positive, congratulate yourself. Your Third Eye will benefit greatly from you trusting yourself again.

Disassociate fear. "I am always right." Say this sentence out loud. What are your first thoughts on this? Are there any negative associations? If so, take these negative associations and reason them out. Are they really valid, or just baseless fears?

Free-write. Free-writing is the act of writing without stopping to think. Take a piece of paper and a pen, and time yourself. Write for two minutes without stopping at all. Don't worry about grammar or spelling. Let your instincts guide you.

Listen closely. If there are currently others in the room with you having a conversation, stop and listen to them. Hear their every word. Is there anything you think is being unsaid?

Crown Chakra

Massage your head. You don't need someone else to do this. Take hold of your head, and apply pressure in circles with your hands.

Be silent. Sit here, be silent, be still, and just listen to the world around you. The Crown is very closely attuned with the senses, so explore them. Make this "quiet time" a part of your normal day.

Utilize indigo or white. These are the colors associated with this chakra, so as usual find clothes, foods and objects in these colors.

Find something inspirational, and do it. Different people have different things that make them feel inspired. Listening to talks from rights campaigners, reading a good story, or just sitting in the garden might be yours. Know what makes you inspired, and do it right now.

How to maintain your chakra balance.

There are several ways you can maintain balance in your chakras, all of which involve adopting a new routine in your daily life. By practicing regular yoga and meditation, as well as implementing other practices, you can help keep your chakras clean and balanced.

Yoga

The practice of yoga began over five thousand years ago, created by an ancient civilization in Northern India. Yoga, as we understand it today, comes from a development of these ancient ideas into what is known as Hatha Yoga. It is beneficial not only for physical fitness but also the fitness of the mind and spirit. Physically, you may find yourself losing weight, improving your immune system, increasing your flexibility, and becoming more energetic. Mentally you may find release from stress, greater intuition, and having better relationships.

Due to its origins, Yoga is crucial to chakra balancing. By making yoga a regular routine in your life, you can help shift the prana around your chakras to balance your chakra system. Each Chakra benefits from a certain asana (yoga pose). It is important to remember that asana can be difficult for a beginner, so always make sure you only do what you are comfortable doing.

For your Root chakra, you might like to try the Vrksasana (or Tree Pose). Stand comfortably, with your feet in line with your hips. As you exhale, loosen your lower half, and slowly raise your right foot, placing it on the inside of your left thigh. Hold this position for five, careful breaths, and then switch sides and repeat. You will be able to feel the prana energy shifting inside you.

For your Sacral chakra, you will feel benefits from the Deviasana (or Goddess Pose). Stand with your feet wide apart pointing away from you, and stoop so your knees come in line with your feet. Place your hands in the center of your thighs, and as you breathe deeply, rhythmically rock your pelvis. This pose is all about feeling the pleasure of the movement, so you should feel free to make any kind of noise you wish. Do this for 8-10 breaths.

For your Solar Plexus chakra, the Navasana (or

Boat Pose) works well. Sit on the floor or ground with your legs out, and place your hands on the surface behind you. Without exhaling, draw your knees towards your chest, and lean back. You are aiming to have a 90° angle between your torso and legs. Then, stretch your legs out as far as you can. Then, extend your arms, and try to touch your lower legs. Maintain this pose for however long you feel comfortable. When you come out, lower your legs to the floor, supporting yourself with your hands behind your back.

For your Heart chakra, try the Ustrasana (or Camel Pose). Whilst on your knees, sit on your heels. With your toes gripping the floor, raise your hips. Place your hands on your hips, and then slowly reach and lean back to hold your feet. Try to have your head and neck parallel with your legs as much as you can. Stay in this pose as long as you feel comfortable. As you come out, straighten your back and sit on your heels, and return your hands to praying position, bowing your head.

For your Throat chakra, there is the option of the Salamba Sarvangasana (or Supported Shoulderstand). Lie down, with a blanket or otherwise soft, raised surface beneath your shoulders. As you bend your knees, lift your legs up. You are aiming to have your legs extended above your head. Support your back with your hands. Hold this pose for two minutes, if you are comfortable. As you release yourself from this pose, return to lying position slowly; vertebrae by vertebrae.

For your Third Eye chakra, you might like to try the Sukhasana (or Easy Pose). Very simply, sit down, making sure your knees are below your hips (use a blanket to sit on if you have to). Bend each knee one at a time, putting your heels to your groin. Hold your hands in front of you, placing your fingertips together. Close your eyes for ten breaths, and ask yourself a question. Concentrate on your breathing. As you inhale, place the tip of your tongue to the roof of your mouth, and release it as you exhale. Place your hands on your knees, and wait to see if you have an answer to your question. You should remain in the Sukhasana for five minutes.

For your Crown chakra, you may try the Savasana (or Corpse Pose). Making sure you are completely comfortable and relaxed, lie down on your back. Keep your feet shoulder-width apart, and extend your arms downwards, and place the palms of your hands faced upwards. As you inhale deeply, tighten your body, letting your head and limbs come up off of the ground or floor. As you exhale, relax. Repeat this for 5-20 minutes.

These are just suggestions of asanas that have great benefits for each chakra; there are many more that you might like to try. By keeping a regular routine of Yoga, using whichever asanas you choose, this can help to maintain balance in your chakras.

Meditation

Meditation is a crucial part of the chakra system. It is used to increase wellbeing, connect with your higher self, relax, and help your physical and mental goodness. By using poses, chanting, and visualizing, meditation can balance an upset chakra effectively. After every meditation, you should feel "clean" in that chakra.

For your Root chakra, first, you must ground yourself. Stand straight with the feet shoulder-width apart. Move your pelvis forward, so that you are completely balanced, then let your weight go forward. Remain like this for several minutes. Then, sit cross-legged, with your left leg over your right leg, with the soles of your feet pointing upwards. Place the tip of your index finger and thumb together on each hand, and relax. Let your hands rest on your knees, with your palms upwards. Visualize your red Toot chakra inside of you, between your genitals and your anus, and think about all it means, and how it affects you and your life, and also how you'd like it to affect you. As you do, chant the word "lam" without vocalizing. Maintain this until you feel completely relaxed.

For your Sacral chakra, sit on your legs with your back upright in a comfortable position. Place your hands on your lap. With your left hand beneath your right, keep your thumbs straight and touch the tips together, letting the fingers of your right hand rest over the fingers of your left hand. Then, visualize your orange Sacral chakra in your lower back, and think about all it means, and how it is affecting you and your life, as well as how you'd like it to. As you do, chant the word "vam" in silence. Maintain this until you feel completely relaxed.

For your Solar Plexus chakra, adopt the same starting position as you would for your Sacral chakra, but with your hands, hold them in front of your stomach and with your elbows bent. Extend your fingers and place your palms together, with your left thumb over your right thumb. Then, visualize the yellow Solar Plexus chakra inside the center of your torso, and everything it means. Silently chant, "ram". Keep thinking about this chakra's effect on you currently, and what you would like it to be until you are relaxed.

For your Heart chakra, adopt the position of the Root chakra, including the shape of the hands. Rest your left hand on your left knee, and your right hand on the center of your chest, with your fingers pointing outwards. Concentrate on everything to do with the Heart chakra, visualizing its green energy inside the center of your chest behind your heart and everything associated with this chakra, including how it currently affects you, and how you'd like it to affect you. Silently chant the word, "yam" as you do this. Keep this pose, chant, and these thoughts until you are relaxed.

For your Throat chakra, adopt the sitting posture of the Sacral chakra. Raise your hands in front of your neck, interlocking your fingers and pressing the tips of your thumbs together, so your nails point towards you, and your thumbs form a pyramid-shape. Concentrate on this blue chakra at the base of your throat, seeing all it represents and how you might currently be feeling from this chakra, as well as what you would like it to do for you. Silently chant, "ham". Keep concentrating until you feel relaxed.

For your Third Eye chakra, sit as you would for your Root chakra. Raise your hands, knuckles together with the thumbs touching tips in front of you. Straighten your middle fingers, keeping the tips together, and point the tips of your thumbs towards you. Visualize the Third Eye chakra inside the center of your head, behind your eyes, thinking about its influence on you and your life, and also how you'd like it to work for you. Without making a sound, chant, "om" or "aum". Keep doing this until you feel completely relaxed.

There are many other ways of maintaining balance in your chakras, so make sure to look into everything, such as Tai Chi, reiki, aromatherapy, acupuncture, and crystal healing. As long as you keep a regular routine, you will feel the positive effects from your balanced chakras.

Your next step towards health and happiness.

Understanding your chakras, knowing how they work, being able to tell if they're imbalanced, and having the ability to rebalance them can help you physically, mentally, and spiritually in many different ways. As explained in chapter one, alongside other systems in the human body, the chakra system is a crucial part of your general wellbeing. Flowing with cosmic energy (prana), your chakras are energy points on your body that help to shape your life. With each chakra working with different parts of your physical being, your mental being and your spiritual being, together the chakras work as part of a whole system. Chakras rely on each other to disperse prana throughout you to keep you healthy and happy.

If you take the time to balance your chakras, you

will reap the benefits — a notion we explored in chapter two. Balancing can result in the strengthening of the immune system, warding off negative emotions and energies. It can help you to control your emotions healthily, and manage them in an appropriate way. You can make sure you have the drive and willpower to succeed in anything you do, whilst having better relationships and connections with those around you. You channel your abilities, increasing your advantages in life. You can avoid negative thought or behavior patterns, by enhancing your self-worth, increasing your confidence, and even giving you the tools to help you overcome addictions or long-term mental health problems. Alongside modern medicine, you can really give yourself a chance. Start living as who you want to be, do what you want to do, and feel what you want to feel.

When the chakras are imbalanced, this can lead to hugely negative thoughts, emotions, behaviors, and even physical ailments. As the chakras are so strongly connected with certain physical areas and mental processes, any imbalance can cause problems. In your body, you could find yourself being constantly ill, in pain, or suffering from some other problem. In your head, you could lose confidence in yourself and in others. You may find your capacity to trust and love plummeting, causing bad relationships with those around you. You could be unable to speak clearly or interpret others. You could become depressed, anxious, or otherwise some long-term mental problem. Your emotions could continuously fluctuate from extreme to extreme—one minute, there's anger, the next, you could be crying. You could become a closed-off, cold person, disconnected from everything.

The seven chakras each govern different aspects of you, explained in chapter three. Not only are they associated with the physical areas around them, but also with parts of your raw emotional and mental template. The Root is your primal instinct; the Sacral is your emotions; the Solar Plexus is your willpower; your Heart is your love; the Throat, communication; the Third Eye, intuition; and the Crown your awareness and wisdom. Knowing how each chakra affects you, makes it much easier to tell which ones may be out of balance. Identifying is usually quite easy, as written in chapter four. Among many other issues, if you're worried about money and being able to provide for your family, the Root chakra is most likely to blame. Being over emotional at anything is an over activity of the Sacral chakra. Having low self-esteem, causing you to hide your ideas from others? The Solar Plexus is to blame. Being too clingy to your partner in a relationship, resulting in you stifling them and worsening things between you? The Heart chakra may be having problems. Finding it difficult to say what you need to say in a presentation? The Throat chakra could be imbalanced. Do you find yourself frequently drifting out of reality, daydreaming, to detrimental amounts? Your Third Eye could be having issues. Are you having problems letting go of an emotion from an event long since gone? Your Crown may be overactive. Once the imbalanced chakra is identified, it is important to remember that an imbalance in one chakra leads to an imbalance of another, and blocked chakras are not mutually exclusive. For example, if you find yourself being overemotional from a badly-delivered presentation, you should take a look at both, your Sacral and your Throat chakras, as well as the ones surrounding them.

As the popularity of chakras grows across the globe, it is beneficial to know that keeping your chakras in balance does not need to be a clinical process. Balancing is not difficult. With the techniques outlined in chapter five, with some simple activities you can do immediately, such as going for a walk or free-writing, you can begin to help your chakras rebalance. Each chakra benefits from a different type of activity, depending on its function in the chakra system. Doing certain activities or utilizing the color the chakra is associated with can be starting steps to helping you redress the balance.

Once the balance has been restored, you can then maintain this with the techniques in chapter six. Incorporating yoga and/or meditation into your daily life will help you to remain in balance. By doing these activities, this will help the chakras stay level, as well as enhancing your meditative or yoga experience. With specific positions and sounds related to each individual chakra, you can take control and nurse each chakra without even leaving the house. Just thirty minutes a day will be enough for you to feel the benefits of these activities.

The details listed in this book are not all you can do to help balance your chakras. Should you wish to explore it, the world of chakras is almost limitless and hugely personal. Certain balancing techniques you may find suits you better than others, and you should explore all options available. Some of these options could be:

Taking a class

There is more than likely a class related to chakras near you. It could be Yoga, Meditation, Tai-Chi or other meditative exercises. There are also classes available, taught by professional healers, to help you understand your chakras even better.

Having aromatherapy

The natural smells of the Earth are also important in chakras, with smells associated with different chakras. You might wish to have a massage by a professional, or you could use them in your living space. You could also use smells in conjunction with meditation, or a meditative exercise. You can also use them directly by rubbing the natural oils on the place of your chakra.

Using reiki

Reiki is the ancient art of putting energy into

someone through massage. This energy, transferred from another person, can help to address any imbalances and maintain a healthy chakra system. To learn more about reiki, go online, or find a reiki practitioner near you. There are also classes available for you to take, so you can use reiki on others who may be having chakra problems.

Crystal healing

Either by consulting a professional or doing it yourself, you can use crystals—natural products from the Earth—to help your chakras. Certain crystals have certain benefits for certain chakras, and you should look into all options. You can use crystals in everyday life, by utilizing their power in a living space, carrying them in your pocket or wearing them, helping you to cope with everyday circumstances.

All of these techniques can be used with each other to help you maintain or heal your chakra balance, and there are many other popular chakra-balancing techniques, too. Remember that you are an individual, and you may find certain techniques work for you better than others, so explore everything you can. Chakra balancing is a long-term pursuit, and you should find yourself willing to learn everything you can. With all of the information in this book, you can manage your cosmic energy in a way that's positive to you, and you can control the way you wish to live your life.